Understanding Fluorescein Angiography

眼底荧光血管造影解析

（中英对照）

〔德〕曼弗雷德·施皮茨纳斯　编著

潘铭东　刘光辉　郑永征　主译

刘晓玲　审校

天津出版传媒集团

天津科技翻译出版有限公司

著作权合同登记号:图字:02-2014-490

图书在版编目(CIP)数据

眼底荧光血管造影解析/(德)施皮茨纳斯(Spitznas,M.)编著;潘铭东等译. —天津:天津科技翻译出版有限公司,2015.6
书名原文:Understanding fluorescein angiography
ISBN 978 - 7 - 5433 - 3478 - 6

Ⅰ.①眼…　Ⅱ.①施…　②潘…　Ⅲ.①眼底荧光摄影 - 研究
Ⅳ.①R770.41

中国版本图书馆 CIP 数据核字(2015)第 046748 号

Translation from English/German/Spanish language edition:
Understanding Fluorescein Angiography, *Fluoreszeinangiografie verstehen*, *Entendiendo Angiografía con Fluoresceína* by Manfred Spitznas
Copyright © 2006 Springer Berlin Heidelberg
Springer Berlin Heidelberg is a part of Springer Science + Business Media

授权单位:Springer-Verlag GmbH
出　　版:天津科技翻译出版有限公司
出 版 人:刘 庆
地　　址:天津市南开区白堤路 244 号
邮政编码:300192
电　　话:(022)87894896
传　　真:(022)87895650
网　　址:www. tsttpc. com
印　　刷:高教社(天津)印务有限公司
发　　行:全国新华书店
版本记录:787×1092　16 开本　8.5 印张　100 千字
　　　　　2015 年 6 月第 1 版　　2015 年 6 月第 1 次印刷
　　　　　定价:68.00 元

译者名单

主　译

潘铭东　福建中医药大学附属人民医院

刘光辉　福建中医药大学附属人民医院

郑永征　福建中医药大学附属人民医院

审　校

刘晓玲　温州医科大学附属眼视光医院

译者前言

眼底荧光血管造影对眼底病的诊断、鉴别诊断、治疗选择、预后推断都具有非常重要的价值，其自 20 世纪 60 年代应用于临床以来，发展迅速，技术日臻完善，成为现代眼科不可缺少的诊断技术。

解读眼底荧光血管造影现象，不仅要求掌握各种眼底疾病的造影特征，还要求熟悉各种造影现象背后所隐藏的机制。Manfred Spitznas 教授的 *Understanding Fluorescein Angiography* 一书正是为此目的而作。该书图文并茂，从光学性、机械性、动态性三个独特的视角解读了眼底荧光血管造影的现象及机制，让人耳目一新。相信该书对眼科医师学习和掌握眼底荧光血管造影读片技术、更准确地诊治眼底疾病大有裨益。

在过去的几个月中，我们在工作之余对原著进行了翻译，希望能将国外眼底荧光血管造影解读的一些理念引入国内，互通有无。期间，承蒙温州医科大学附属眼视光医院刘晓玲教授在百忙之中对翻译工作进行了指导，并审阅了全部译稿，在此表示衷心的感谢。

由于编译时间仓促，译者经验不足、水平有限，翻译的谬误之处在所难免，恳请各位专家、同道、读者不吝赐教，对译文的纰漏和错误之处作出指正。

2015 年 1 月 20 日于吉祥山

前　言

　　荧光血管造影是现代眼科不可缺少的工具。

　　通过静脉注射荧光素钠进入眼底组织,并观察相关现象,荧光血管造影为眼科医生提供了宝贵的诊断信息。

　　本书介绍了荧光血管造影下的组织形态特征及结构性改变。

Preface

Fluorescein angiography is an indispensable tool in modern ophthalmology.

It is based on the behavior of intravenously administered sodium fluorescein in the tissues of the ocular fundus. The phenomena observed provide the ophthalmologist with valuable diagnostic information.

This book describes the morphological characteristics and structural changes underlying these phenomena.

目　录

Contents

第 1 章

基本要点

Basic facts

Chapter 1

正常中央视网膜毛细血管

❯ 荧光血管造影是一项不同寻常的活体检查技术，其能够显示黄斑中心凹无血管区(foveal avascular zone, FAZ)旁周管径仅 3.5μm 的微小毛细血管(图 1 上)——该血管管径约为红细胞直径的一半大小。

由于 FAZ 旁周的毛细血管管径微细，红细胞必须改变形态才能通过，于是需占据更多的血管腔空间，从而使该区域血管不能由全血灌注(图 1 下)。

Normal central retinal capillaries

❯ Fluorescein angiography is a remarkable *in vivo* technique, because it is able to resolve the minute capillaries in the neighborhood of the foveal avascular zone which measure only 3.5 μm in diameter (*top*). This is half the diameter of red blood cells.

Because of their small diameter, the capillaries in the vicinity of the foveal avascular zone cannot be perfused with whole blood, since the red blood cells have to change their shape in order to pass, thus requiring much more space (*bottom*).

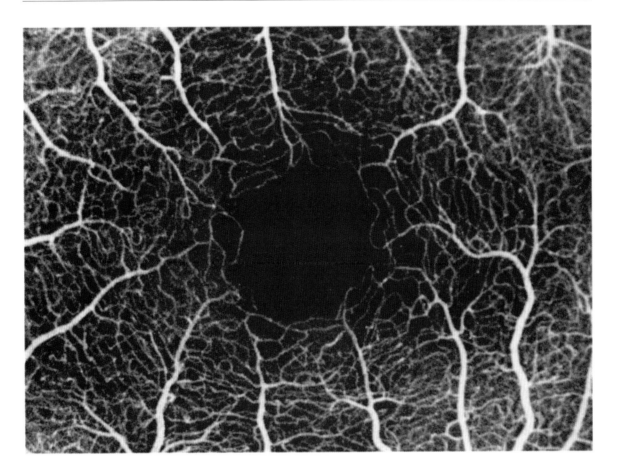

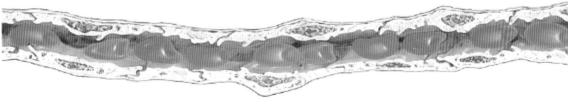

图 1

正常周边视网膜毛细血管

❯ 在远离 FAZ 的视网膜血管中,细胞浓度升高。这些富集的细胞中的大部分通常可能通过视网膜远周部广泛的血管网(分流毛细血管)进入静脉。视网膜远周部的这些毛细血管在紧邻锯齿缘处形成长短不一的回路(长,图 2 上;短,图 2 中)。它们的管腔最宽可达 20 μm(图 2 下)。

Normal peripheral retinal capillaries

❯ The cell concentration in the retinal vessels further away from the foveal avascular zone is increased. The bulk of surplus cells is most likely transported to the venous side by wide vascular channels, so-called *shunt capillaries*, in the far periphery of the retina. These capillaries form long (*top*) or short (*middle*) loops in the immediate vicinity of the ora serrata. Their lumen is up to 20 μm wide (*bottom*).

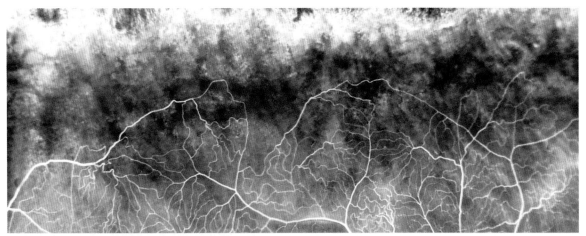

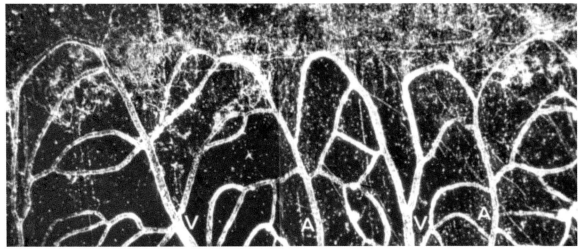

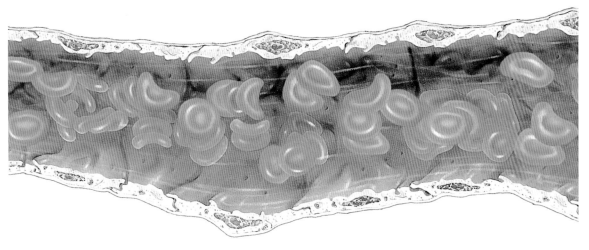

图 2

阻塞的周边视网膜毛细血管

❯❯ 分流毛细血管可因为以下原因而出现阻塞(图3上):

1.红细胞丧失变形能力(镰状细胞贫血);

2.红细胞数量显著增加(居于高海拔地区,红细胞增多症);

3.管壁增厚致管腔变窄(Eales 病)。

上述 3 种原因可以导致周边视网膜缺氧,继而出现新生血管(图 3 下)。

Plugged peripheral retinal capillaries

❯❯ The shunt capillaries can become *plugged* (*top*) due to

1. loss of deformability of red blood cells (sickle cell disease)

2. further increase of red blood cells (living at high altitude, polycythemia)

3. narrowing of vascular lumen due to wall thickening (Eales' disease)

Thc result in all three instances is peripheral hypoxia followed by neovascularization (*bottom*).

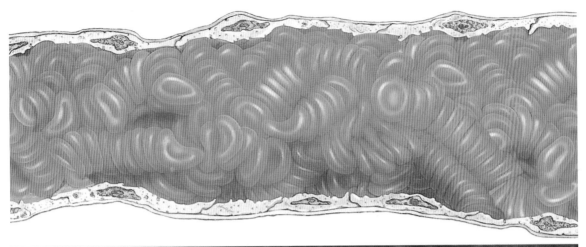

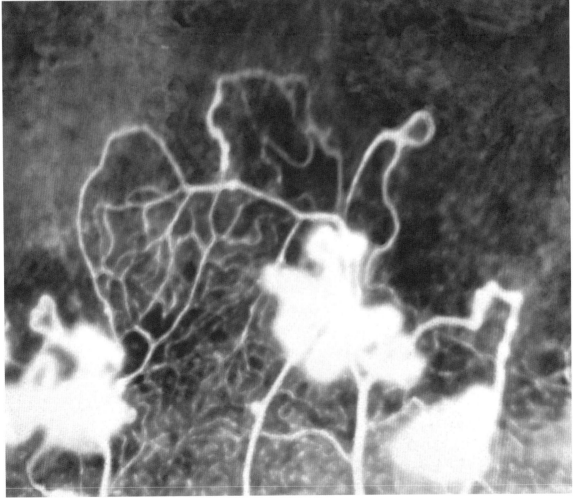

图 3

> 荧光血管造影现象可以从以下 3 个方面进行解读：

- 光学性
- 机械性
- 动态性

> The phenomena of fluorescein angiography are divided into

- optical
- mechanical
- dynamic

第 2 章

光学现象

Optical phenomena

Chapter 2

光学现象

与眼部组织的透明性相关,透明性可表现为:

- 正常
- 减弱
- 增强

Optical phenomena

are related to the *transparency* of ocular tissues. Transparency may be

- normal
- decreased
- increased

神经视网膜的透明性

> **神经视网膜为透明组织。**

因此,下方脉络膜的染色——背景荧光变得可见。在明亮染色的视网膜血管的衬托下,背景荧光呈弥漫性灰霾样(图 4)。

Transparency of neurosensory retina

> **The neurosensory retina is transparent.**

For this reason the so-called background fluorescence, i.e. the staining of the underlying choroids, becomes visible. It appears as a diffuse gray haze behind much brighter stained retinal vessels.

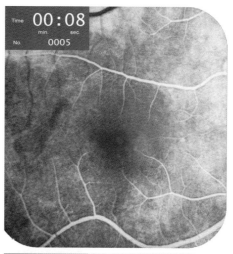

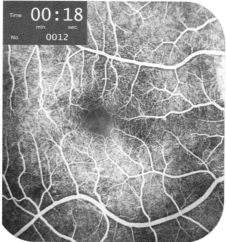

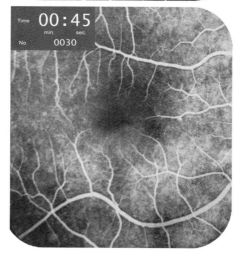

图 4

正常

透明结构

▶ 即使神经视网膜由多层组成,其仍惊人地透明。虽然在显微镜下其细胞核层深染,但是这似乎并不影响其透明性(图5)。事实上,这一现象是符合逻辑的,因为呈现在眼前的图像在进入光感受器单元之前必须经过神经视网膜的所有亚层。

星号=光感受器

Normal

Transparent structures

▶ The transparency of the neurosensory retina is surprising since it is composed of so many layers. But even the nuclei that stain dark under the microscope do not seem to interfere with transparency. In fact, this is logical because the image that is presented to the eye has to travel through all these layers before reaching the receptor elements.

asterisk = photoreceptors

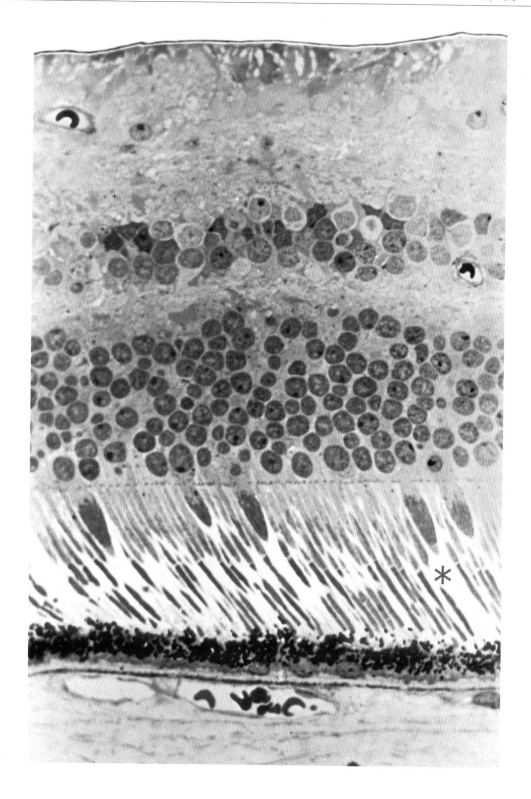

图 5

减弱

死亡后

❯ 人死亡后，视网膜因为水肿而丧失其透明性，呈白色，黄斑区的黄色素亦因此变得可见——在正常的情况下是不可见的。

图 6 为经墨水灌注的尸体眼。

Decreased

Post mortem

❯ After death, the retina loses its transparency due to *edema* and turns white so that the *yellow macular pigment*, which is normally invisible, can be seen.

cadaver eye perfused with ink

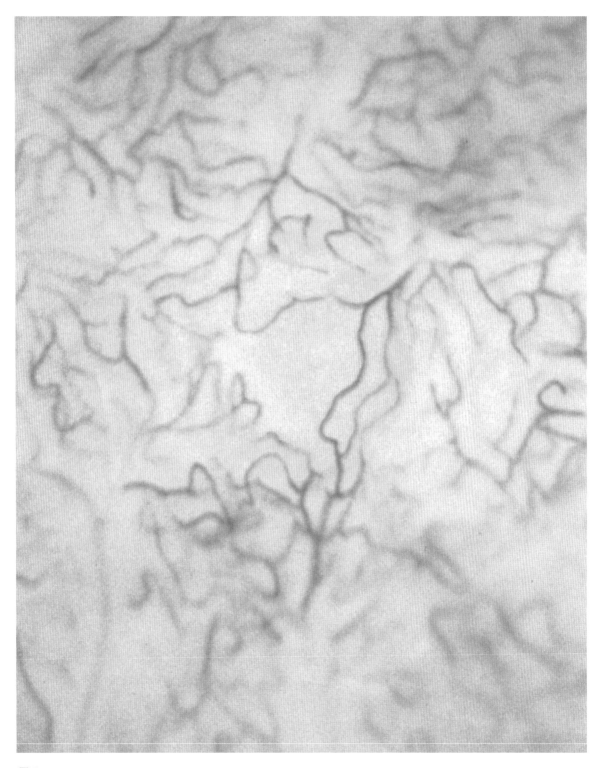

图 6

血液

> 在活体眼中,视网膜水肿可见于一系列病理改变,其在荧光血管造影中可遮蔽正常的脉络膜背景荧光(如下例图片所示)。

图 7 为晚期糖尿病视网膜病变的水肿。

Blood

> In the living eye, *edema* that obscures the normal background fluorescence of the choroid in the fluorescein angiogram can occur under a variety of pathological conditions as illustrated with this case.

edema in advanced diabetic retinopathy

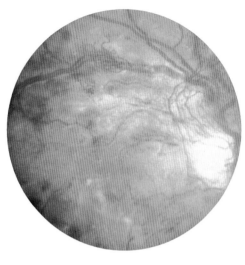
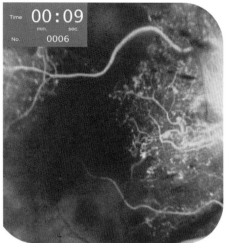
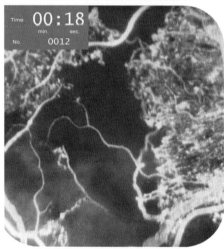
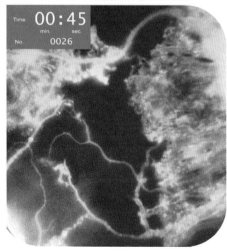

图 7

▶ 视网膜完全丧失透明性及相应的脉络膜背景荧光湮灭常常由于出血所致(图 8)。当出血的累积量大时,其很容易被识别。

▶ Total loss of retinal transparency and, with it, choroidal background fluorescence, is usually caused by *blood*. When accumulations of blood are large, they are easy to recognize.

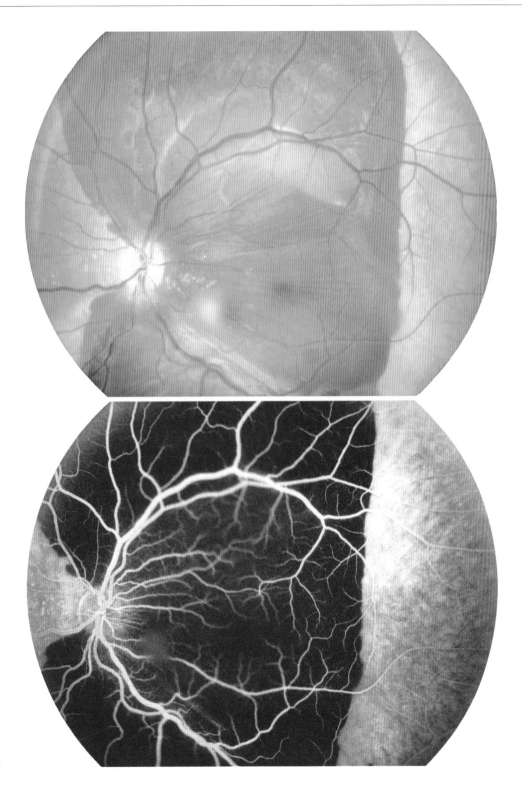

图 8

> 小的出血灶也能遮蔽脉络膜背景荧光,呈低荧光暗区。当出血呈多灶性或者位于中心凹外时,其也很容易被识别(图9)。

> *Small hemorrhages* also obscure background choroidal fluorescence and thus appear dark. When they are multiple and located outside the foveola, they are easily recognized.

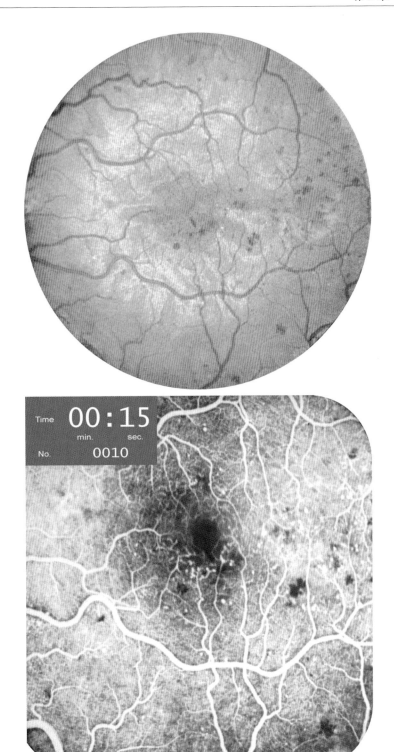

图 9

❱ 中心凹区的小出血灶(图 10 上)容易被忽略,或误读为正常 FAZ(图 10 下)。因此,视网膜中央区的血管造影片一般需要放大审阅。

❱ Small hemorrhages located in the area of the fovea (*top*) are easily overlooked or mistaken for the normal foveal avascular zone (*bottom*). For this reason, angiograms of the central retina should always be viewed under magnification.

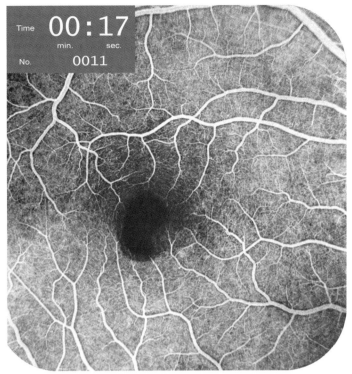

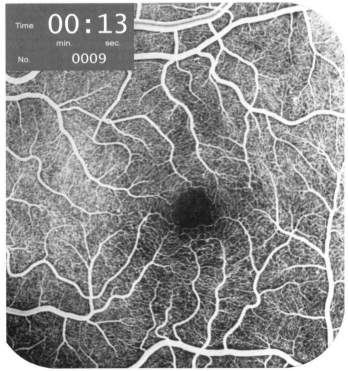

图 10

黑色素

❯ 色素的积聚也可以导致视网膜透明性的丧失,如本例黑色素细胞瘤(图 11 左)。当色素位于视网膜深层时,仅遮蔽脉络膜背景荧光;当其位置更浅表时,也可以遮蔽视网膜血管荧光。

色素还可以位于视网膜血管壁上或血管内(图 11 右),导致视网膜血管呈节段性不透明,以致于相应位置的荧光血流柱不可见。

Melanin

❯ Accumulations of *pigment* as in this case of melanocytoma (*left*) may also lead to a loss of transparency. When the pigment is located deep in the retina, only choroidal fluorescence is blocked. When it is located more superficially, the retinal vessels are obscured, too.

Pigment can also be present on, or within, the wall of retinal vessels (*right*), making them focally non-transparent so that the fluorescein-stained blood column is no longer visible.

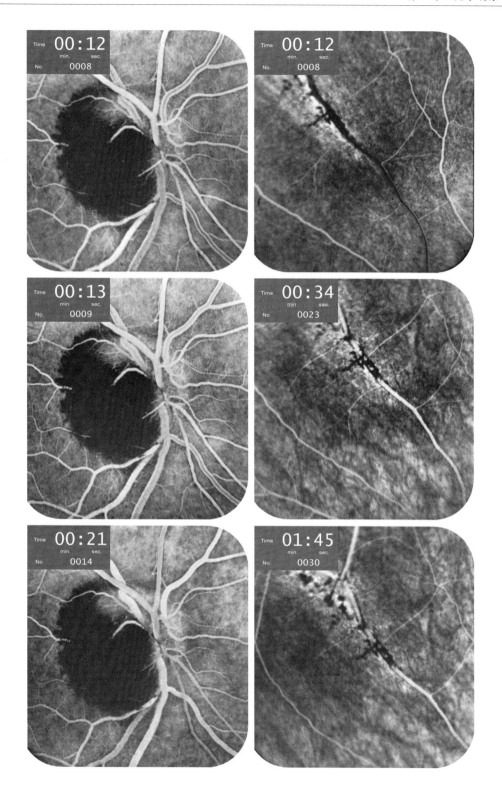

图 11

RPE 的透明性

> **视网膜色素上皮(retinal pigment epithelium, RPE)为半透明性。**

因此,脉络膜背景荧光呈灰暗模糊样(图 12)。

Transparency of retinal pigment epithelium

> **The retinal pigment epithelium is semi-transparent.**

For this reason the background choroidal fluorescence is gray and fuzzy.

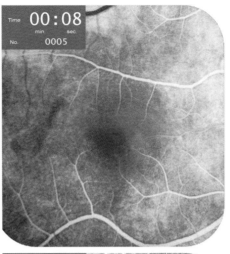

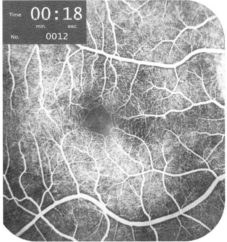

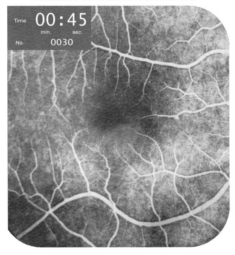

图 12

正常

黑色素颗粒

> 黑色素颗粒影响了色素上皮的透明性(图 13 上)。
>
> 黑色素颗粒越密集的区域,透明性越低,反之亦然(图 13 下)。

箭头=透明性增强的区域

Normal

Melanin granules

> Full transparency is prevented by the presence of *melanin granules* (*top*).
>
> Where these granules are more concentrated the transparency decreases, and vice versa (*bottom*).

arrow = area of increased transparency

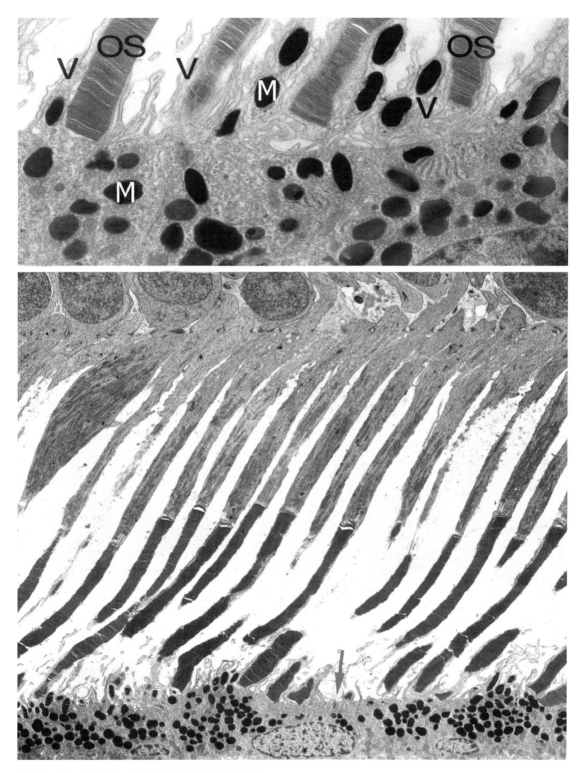

图 13 （注：本书所有图中缩写的解释见书后附表。）

减弱

黄斑

> 由于中心凹及其附近区域的色素上皮细胞密度大,色素含量高,故中心凹区的脉络膜背景荧光远远低于其周围的视网膜(图 14)。

Decreased

Macula

> Background choroidal fluorescence in the fovea is always less pronounced than in the more peripheral retina, because the pigment epithelial cells in, and around, the fovea are higher and contain more pigment than elsewhere.

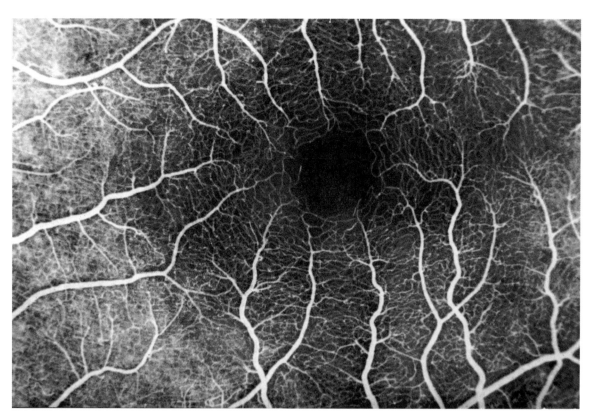

图 14

RPE 肥大

❯ RPE 细胞肥大可完全遮蔽脉络膜背景荧光(图 15)。

Hypertrophy of RPE

❯ *Hypertrophy of the retinal pigment epithelium* totally blocks background choroidal fluorescence.

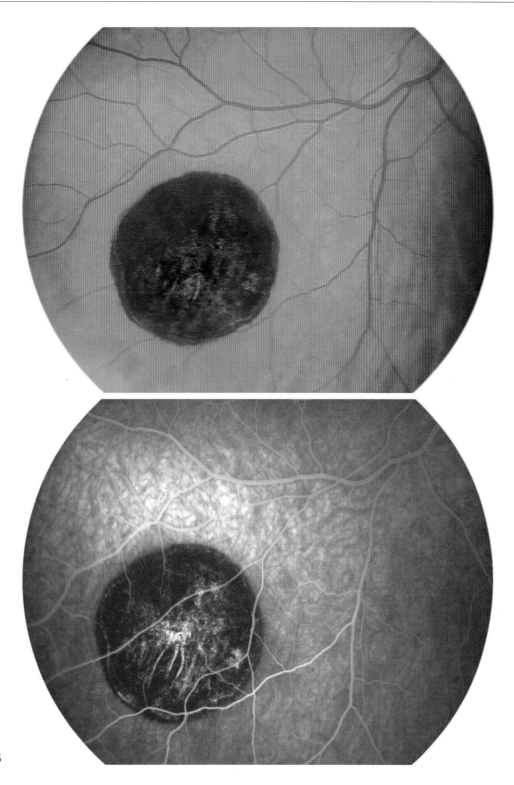

图 15

脉络膜皱褶

❯ 在脉络膜皱褶区,切面图显示在皱褶的斜面多个色素上皮细胞重叠,使这些区域丧失了透明性,呈线状荧光暗区(图 16)。

Choroidal folds

❯ In the region of *choroidal folds*, the tangential view through several superimposed pigment epithelial cells on the slopes of the folds leads to a loss of transparency in these areas, creating the impression of dark stripes.

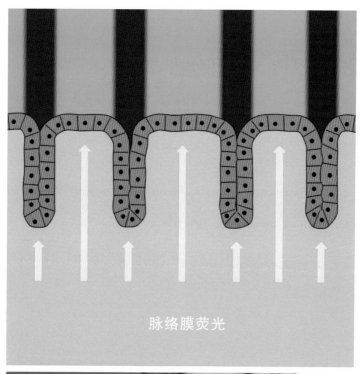

脉络膜荧光

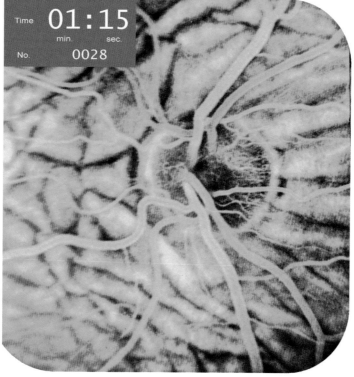

图 16

脉络膜痣

❯ 当色素痣位于脉络膜表层时,如紧邻 Bruch 膜,也能遮蔽脉络膜背景荧光(图 17)。

Choroidal nevi

❯ Background choroidal fluorescence can also be obscured by *nevi* when these are located rather superficially in the choroid, i.e. close to Bruch's membrane.

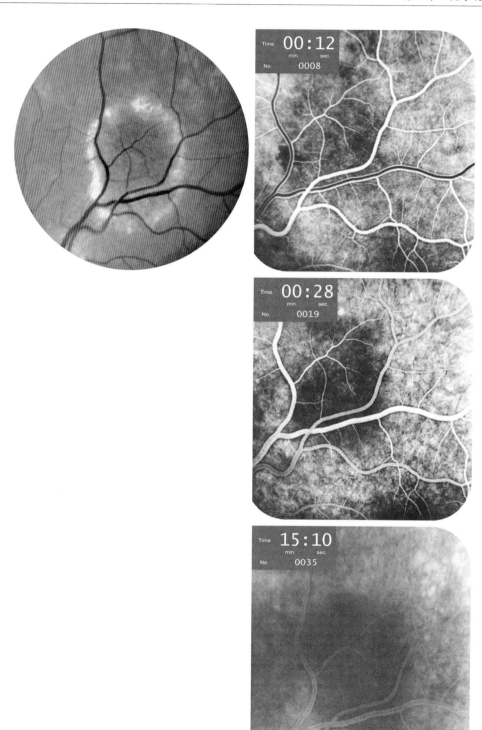

图 17

增强

玻璃疣

❱ 在病理情况下,RPE 的透明性也可以增强。例如,玻璃膜疣之类的透明性物质积聚于色素上皮下时,可引起色素上皮变薄及局灶性色素颗粒稀疏(图 18 上)。这种情况下将出现窗样缺损,产生透见脉络膜荧光。

沿图中(图 18 上)虚线所示做单个玻璃膜疣的水平切面电镜片。图中(图 18 下)环形代表色素上皮基底膜。环外为 RPE 的基底内褶。环内为玻璃膜疣,由透明碎片充斥。

Increased

Drusen

❱ Under pathological conditions the transparency of the retinal pigment epithelium can also be increased. This is the case when transparent materials, such as *drusen*, accumulate under the pigment epithelium, causing thinning of the epithelium and focal dispersion of pigment granules(*top*). In this way a window is formed that allows an unhindered view of choroidal fluorescence.

Electron microscopic flat section (*bottom*) through a single druse along the dotted line in the *top* figure. The ring represents the pigment epithelial basement membrane. Outside are the basal infoldings of the RPE. Inside the ring is the druse, which is filled with transparent debris.

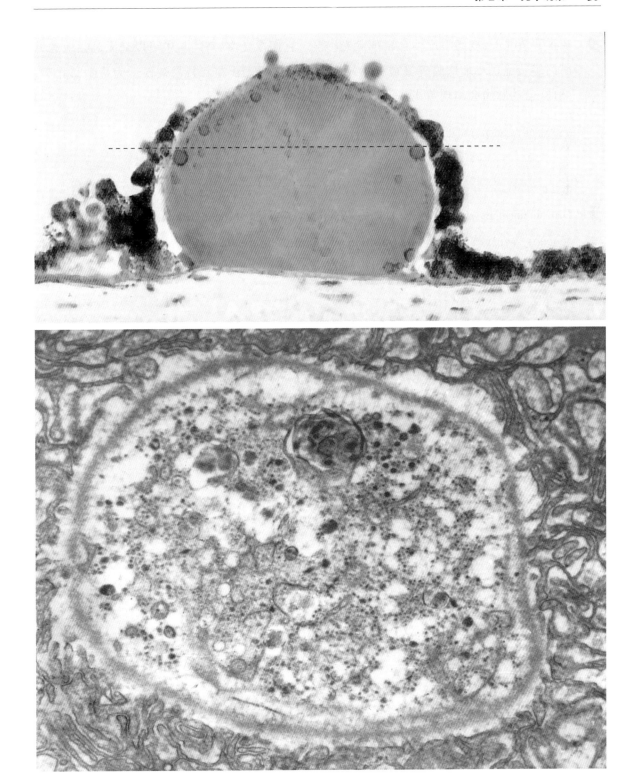

图 18

❱ 在正常情况下,玻璃膜疣不会出现荧光渗漏。它们像光窗一样,从中可以毫无遮拦地透见脉络膜荧光。小玻璃膜疣又被称为硬性玻璃膜疣(图 19 左),其易被误认为是微动脉瘤。然而,微动脉瘤会出现荧光渗漏而玻璃膜疣不会。

左=硬性玻璃膜疣,右=软性玻璃膜疣

❱ Drusen normally *do not leak*. They are optical windows through which the choroidal fluorescence is seen in an unhindered fashion. When drusen are small, so-called hard drusen (*left*), they may be mistaken for microaneurysms; however, microaneurysms leak and drusen do not leak.

left = hard drusen, right = soft drusen

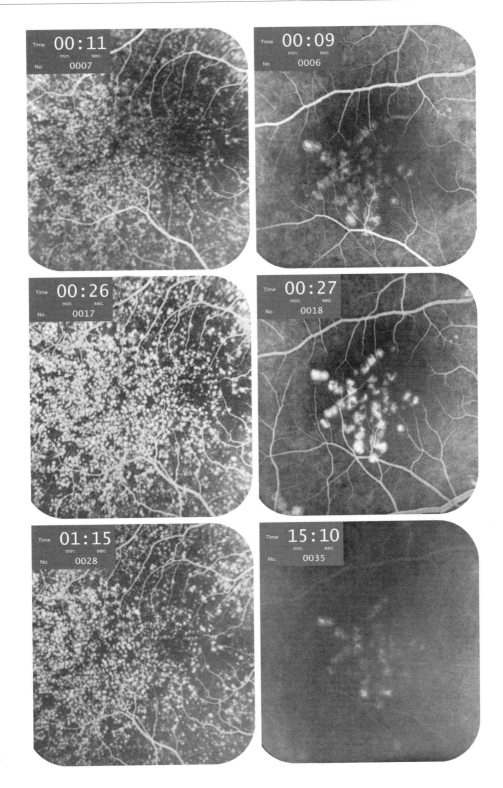

图 19

瘢痕、退行性病变

❯ RPE 瘢痕或者变性（图 20 左）可导致色素紊乱，并使病变区域呈现高、低相间的不均匀荧光。

完全无色素，如网状变性（图 20 右），可使下方脉络膜血管完全显影，并显示其典型着染特征。

Scars, degenerative processes

❯ Scars and degenerative processes in the retinal pigment epithelium (*left*) can lead to pigment mottling with alternating areas of *hyper-and hypofluorescence*.

Total absence of pigment, as in *areolar degeneration* (*right*), provides full visualization of the underlying choroidal vasculature with its typical staining characteristics.

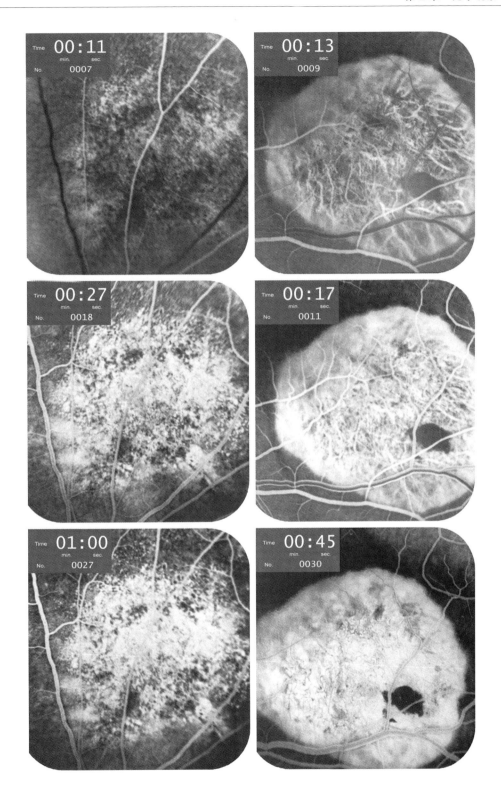

图 20

Bruch 膜的透明性

> Bruch 膜为半透明性(图 21)。

Transparency of Bruch's membrane

> Bruch's membrane is semi-transparent.

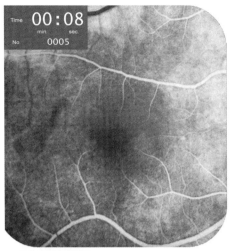

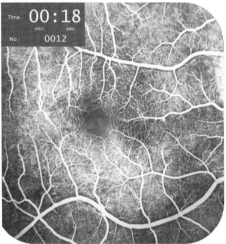

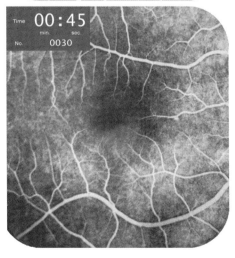

图 21

正常

弹力层

▶ 在光镜(图 22 上)或电镜(图 22 下)下观察 Bruch 膜垂直切片,其中央的弹力层格外清晰,呈一相当实性的结构。

箭头=弹力层

Normal

Elastic layer

▶ When viewed in perpendicular sections under the light microscope (*top*) or electron microscope (*bottom*), especially the elastic *layer* in the center of Bruch's membrane seems to be a rather solid structure.

arrows = elastic layer

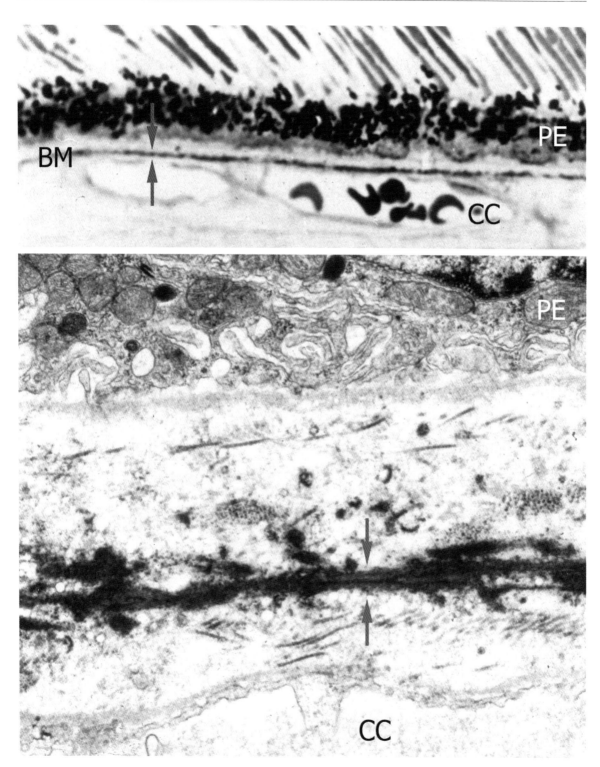

图 22

❯ 但是,无论是在光镜(图 23 上)还是电镜(图 23 下)下,水平铺片都明确显示 Bruch 膜的弹力层绝不是实性结构,而是呈网状结构。因此,Bruch 膜也绝非一个弥漫性的荧光屏障,对其下方脉络膜背景荧光的遮挡相当轻微。

❯ On flat sections it becomes apparent even under the light microscope (*top*) and also under the electron microscope (*bottom*) that the elastic layer of Bruch´s membrane is by no means solid, but open like a sieve. For this reason it does not constitute a diffusion barrier and its interference with the background fluorescence of the underlying choroid is only slight.

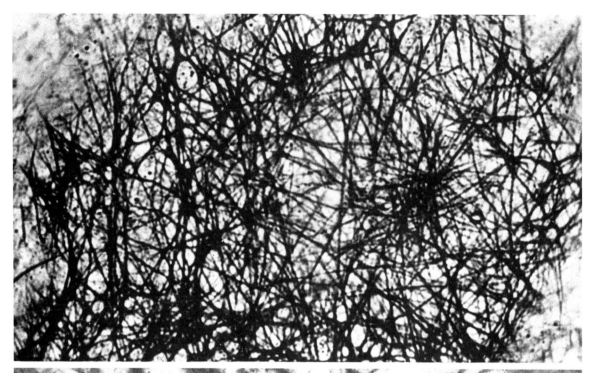

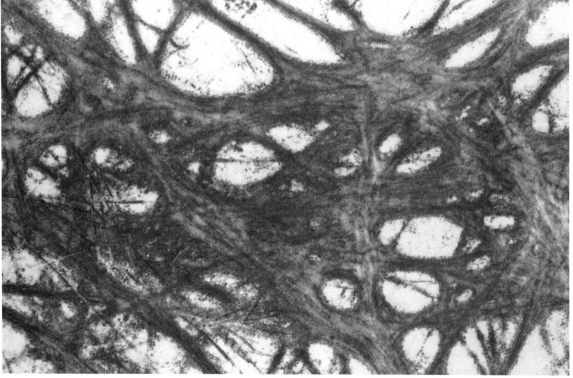

图 23

增强

血管条纹样征

❱ 在血管样条纹症中,Bruch 膜裂开,脉络膜背景荧光的可见度增加,但无荧光渗漏(图 24)。

Increased

Angioid streaks

❱ In *angioid streaks* a dehiscence of Bruch's membrane increases the visibility of choroidal fluorescence and does not show any sign of leakage.

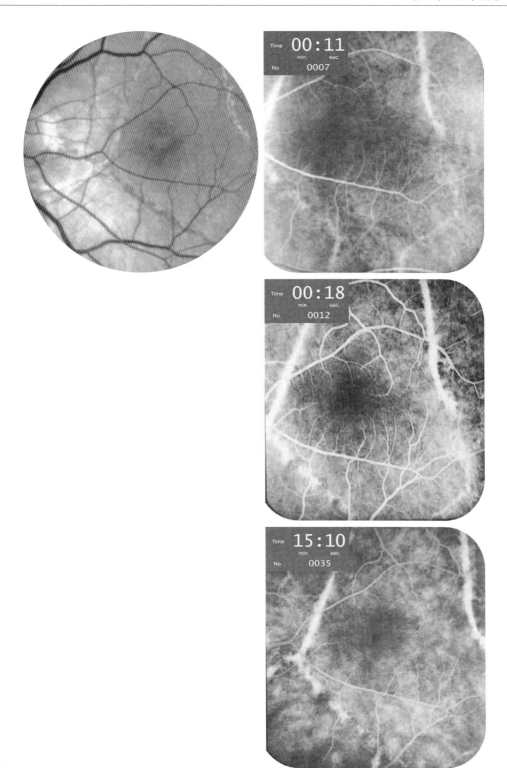

图 24

第3章

机械现象

Mechanical phenomena

Chapter 3

机械现象

与 RPE 对 Bruch 膜的黏附性相关。

Mechanical phenomena

are related to the ***adhesion*** of the retinal pigment epithelium to Bruch's membrane.

RPE 黏附性

> **RPE 与 Bruch 膜连接紧密。**

因此,RPE 通常不会出现泡样改变(图 25)。

Attachment of retinal pigment epithelium

> **The retinal pigment epithelium is firmly attached.**

For this reason the retinal pigment epithelium does not usually form *blisters*.

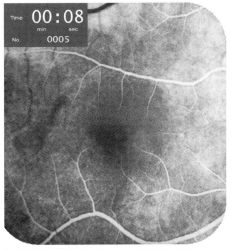

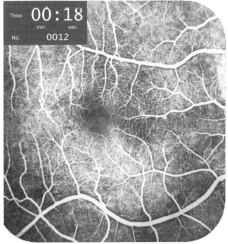

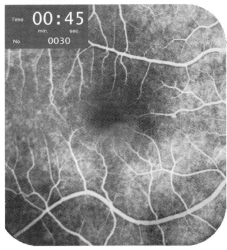

图 25

正常

半桥粒

❯ RPE 通过 RPE 细胞基底侧的半桥粒黏附于 Bruch 膜(图 26 上)。

在电镜下,半桥粒呈细小的黑色致密物,位于色素上皮基底内褶顶端。其具有钉子样功能,能使色素上皮固定于 Bruch 膜(图 26 下)。

箭头=半桥粒

Normal

Hemidesmosomes

❯ The attachment of the retinal pigment epithelium to Bruch's membrane is achieved by the presence of so-called *hemidesmosomes* on the basal side of RPE cells (*top*).

Under the electron microscope the hemidesmosomes are recognized as little black densities at the tips of the basal infoldings of the pigment epithelium. They have the function of tacks that hold the pigment epithelium to Bruch's membrane (*bottom*).

arrows = hemidesmosomes

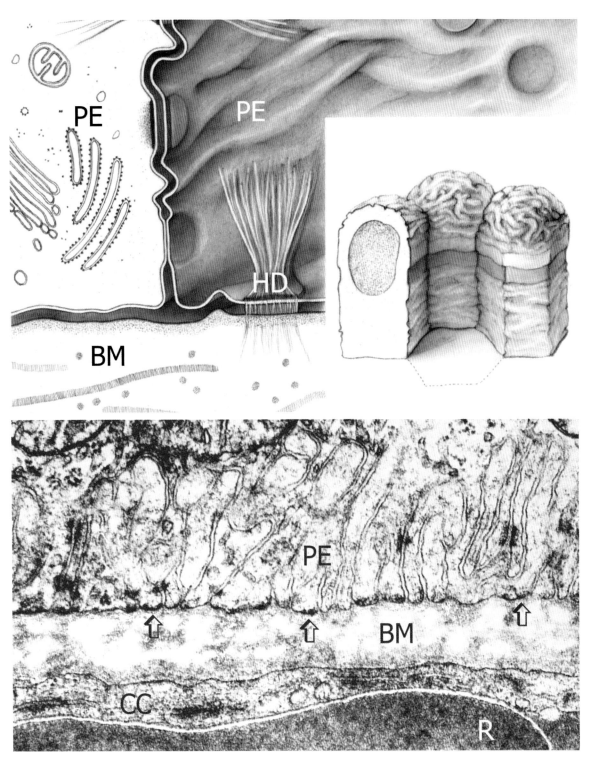

图 26

紊乱

色素上皮脱离

❯ 局灶性半桥粒缺失使 RPE 从 Bruch 膜分离,因此荧光素可以积聚在两者之间(图 27)。在年轻的成年患者中,这种情况被称为Ⅱ型中心性浆液性脉络膜视网膜病变(central serous chorioretinopathy,CSC)。

Disturbed

Pigment epithelial detachment

❯ A focal absence of hemidesmosomes allows the retinal pigment epithelium to split away from Bruch's membrane so that fluorescein-stained fluid can accumulate between them. In young adults this condition is also called *central serous chorioretinopathy type* Ⅱ.

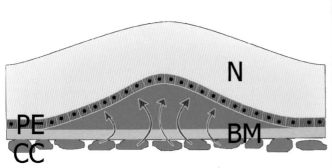

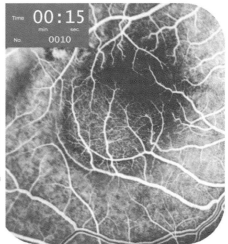

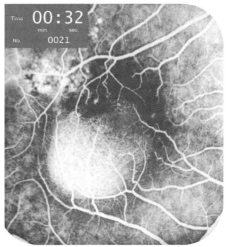

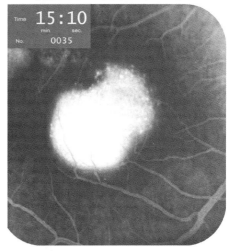

图 27

第 4 章

动态现象

Dynamic phenomena

Chapter 4

动态现象

与荧光素在眼组织中的扩散相关。这种扩散取决于视网膜和脉络膜血管的血－视网膜屏障。

Dynamic phenomena

relate to the diffusion of fluorescein in the ocular tissues. This diffusion is determined by the *blood-retinal barrier* of both the *retinal* and *choroidal vessels*.

形态学与生理学基础

> 荧光素的迁移遵循扩散的基本原则。扩散是指液体或气体分子从高浓度区域向低浓度区域的分子运动。和其他组织一样,视网膜和脉络膜也是由细胞和细胞间隙组成。通常,细胞间隙是荧光素扩散的常规通道,而细胞则构成屏障以抵挡荧光素的自由扩散。然而,这一规则有两个重要的例外,一是毛细血管微孔,二是闭锁小带(图 28)。

红横杠=扩散屏障

Morphologic and physiologic basis

> The migration of fluorescein follows the rules of diffusion. Diffusion is the movement of molecules in liquids or gases from regions of high concentration to regions of low concentration. Like all other tissues the retina and the choroid are composed of *cells* and *intercellular spaces*. In general, intercellular spaces represent the regular pathways for the diffusion of fluorescein, while the cells form a barrier against the free diffusion of fluorescein; however, there are two important exceptions to this rule. One exception is the so-called *capillary pores*; the other is the so-called *zonulae occludentes*.

red bars = diffusion obstacles

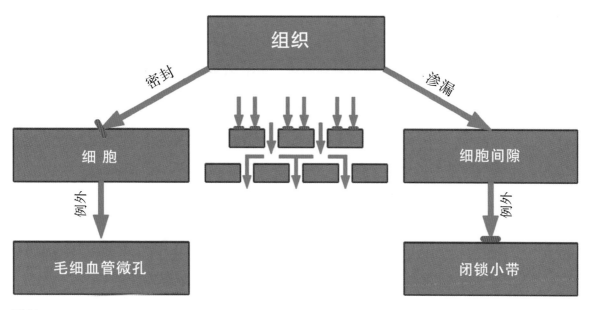

图 28

毛细血管微孔、闭锁小带

❯ 尽管毛细血管微孔(图 29 上)是内皮细胞的一部分,且被部分细胞膜所覆盖,但是其允许荧光素的扩散。

闭锁小带(图 29 下)是细胞间隙的特殊结构,即细胞间连接。相邻细胞的细胞膜在此相互融合,将细胞间隙关闭,阻止扩散。

Capillary pores, zonulae occludentes

❯ Even though *capillary pores* (*top*) are part of endothelial cells and are covered by portions of the cytoplasmic membrane, they allow the diffusion of fluorescein.

Zonulae occludentes (*bottom*) are specialized structures of the intercellular space, so-called intercellular junctions. In their region the cell membranes of the neighboring cells are fused, thus closing the intercellular space and preventing diffusion.

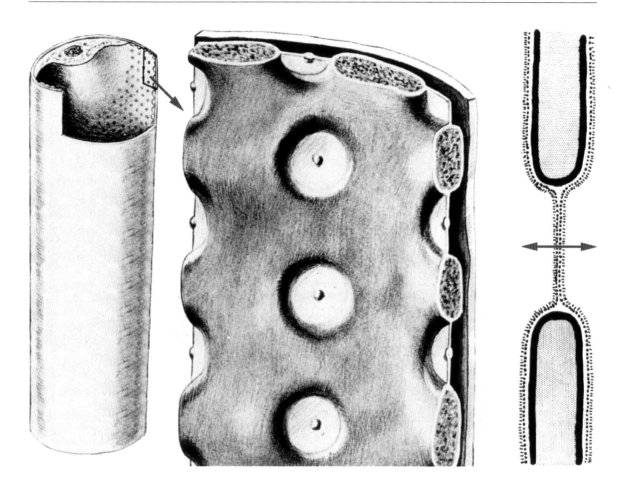

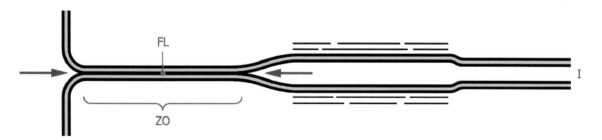

图 29

视网膜血管的渗透性

> **正常视网膜血管对荧光素不通透。**

换句话说,正常视网膜血管是"密封"的。

这主要是因为视网膜毛细血管管腔内衬连续的内皮细胞。而视网膜毛细血管的内皮细胞不存在细胞微孔,细胞间隙也被闭锁小带关闭(图 30)。

Permeability of retinal vessels

> **Normal retinal vessels are non-permeable to fluorescein.**

In other words, normal retinal vessels are "*tight*".

This phenomenon is based on the fact that the lumen of the retinal capillaries is lined by a continuous layer of endothelial cells. The endothelial cells of the retinal capillaries do not carry pores and the intercellular spaces are closed by zonulae occludentes.

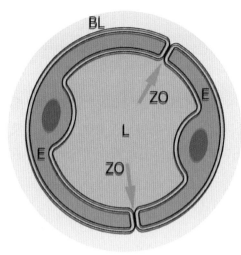

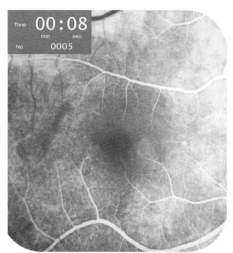

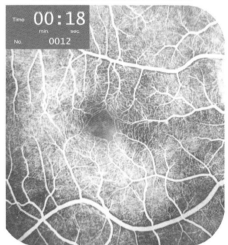

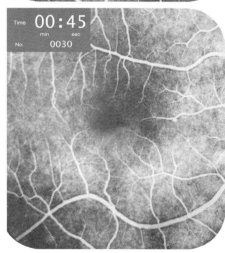

图 30

正常

闭锁小带

❯ 电镜显示一视网膜毛细血管(图 31 右上),中央为管腔,由连续的无微孔的内皮细胞层包绕。右下图为内皮细胞的细胞间隙示例图,闭锁小带在电镜下呈黑色。在顶端及底部细胞间隙呈开放状态,而中间部分细胞间隙由闭锁小带关闭,因此阻止了荧光素的通过。

Normal

Zonulae occludentes

❯ Electron microscopy shows a retinal capillary (*above right*) with its lumen in the center, surrounded by an uninterrupted layer of endothelial cells without pores. *Below* is an example of an intercellular space between endothelial cells. The region of a zonula occludens appears black under the electron microscope. The intercellular space is open in its apical and basal portion, while the central portion is closed by the zonula occludens, thus preventing the passage of fluorescein.

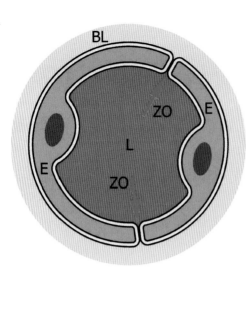

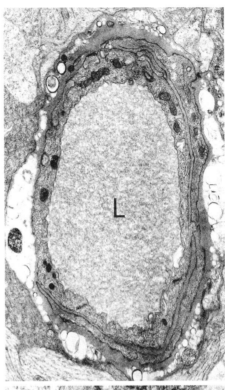

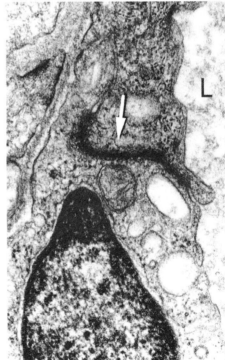

图 31

病理性

❯ 病理状态下,视网膜血管可变得通透,换句话说,它们变得"漏水"了。

视网膜血管在下列情况下出现渗漏:
- 闭锁小带开放(图 32 上);
- 内皮细胞丢失,使得内皮细胞内衬不完整(图 32 中);
- 内皮细胞出现微孔(图 32 下)。

箭头=荧光素渗漏的窗口

Pathologic

❯ *Pathologically*, retinal vessels may become permeable. In other words, they become "*leaky*".

Retinal vessels leak
- when zonulae occludentes *open up* (*top*),
- when endothelial cells are lost, rendering the *endothelial lining incomplete* (*middle*), or
- when the endothelial cells develop pores (*bottom*).

arrows = ports of fluorescein leakage

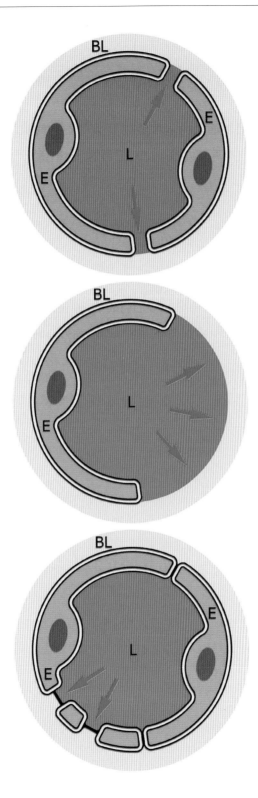

图 32

闭锁小带开放

❯ 典型的闭锁小带开放常出现在炎症性的病例中。

在视网膜血管炎中,荧光素通过内皮细胞间开放的细胞间隙漏出(图33)。荧光着染了病变的血管壁及邻近组织,由此也产生了一个"错误"的术语——"血管周围炎"。

Open zonulae occludentes

❯ Opening of zonulae occludentes is typically the case in *inflammatory conditions*.

In retinal vasculitis fluorescein leaks through the open intercellular spaces of the endothelium. It stains the walls and the vicinity of the diseased vessel and gives rise to the erroneous term "perivasculitis".

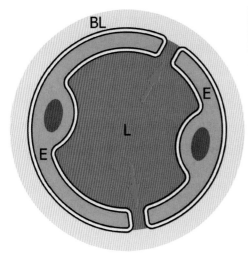

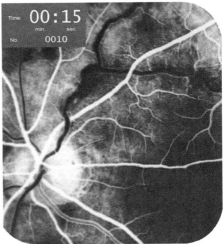

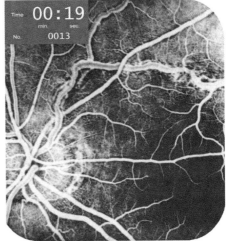

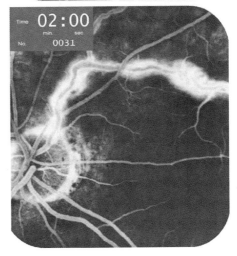

图 33

❯ 图 34 为另外两例视网膜血管炎性荧光渗漏。左侧为多发性硬化,右侧为后葡萄膜炎。渗漏的典型体征表现为受累的血管管径呈节段性扩张。

❯ Two more cases depict the leakage of fluorescein out of inflamed retinal vessels. The underlying disease is multiple sclerosis (*left*) and posterior uveitis (*right*). As a typical feature of leakage, the diseased portions of the vessels seem to grow in diameter.

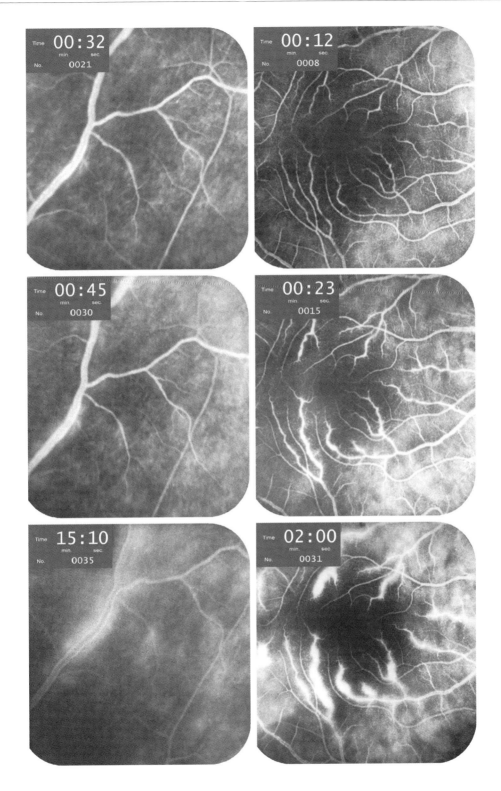

图 34

内皮细胞丧失

❯ 糖尿病微动脉瘤的荧光渗漏通常由内皮细胞丧失所引起(图 35)。

Endothelial cell loss

❯ Leakage out of *diabetic microaneurysms* is usually caused by a loss of endothelial cells.

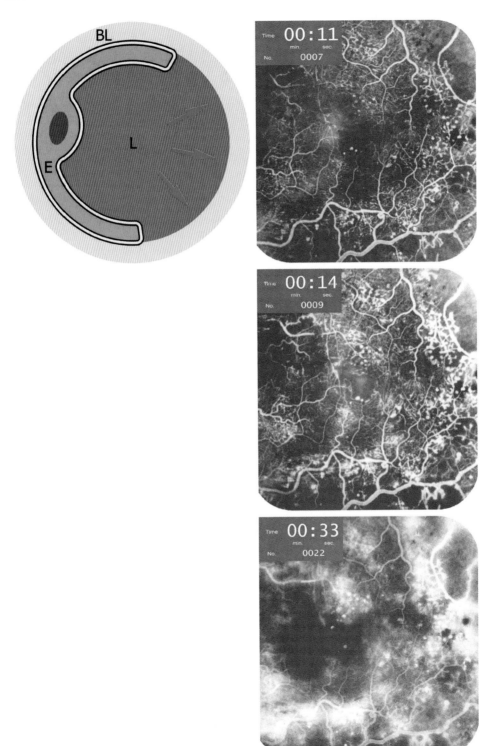

图 35

微孔

> 来自于增殖性视网膜血管的荧光渗漏非常显著,这是由于内皮细胞出现微孔(图 36 左上)
> 及内皮细胞内衬不完整(图 36 左中)所致。

Pores

> Leakage of fluorescein from *proliferated retinal vessels* is very pronounced. It is caused by both
> the occurrence of pores (*left top*) and an incomplete endothelial lining (*left middle*).

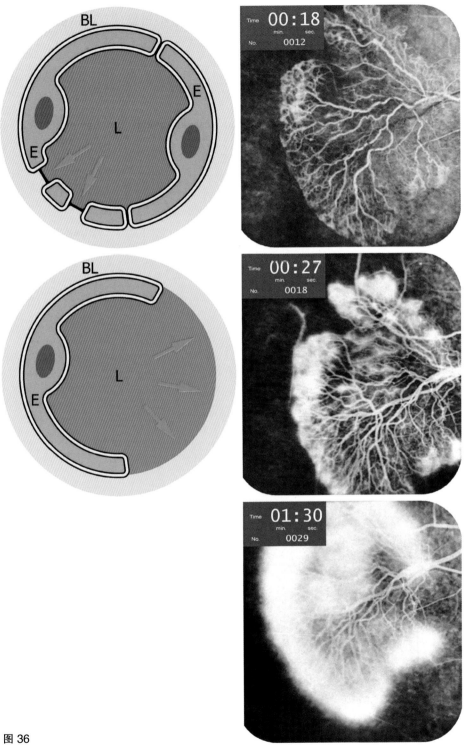

图 36

▶ 增殖性视网膜血管的电镜检查显示内皮细胞内衬不完整(图 37 白箭头)和内皮细胞微孔 (图 37 黑箭头)。

▶ Electron microscopy of proliferated retinal vessels reveals the incomplete endothelial lining (*white arrows*) and pores (*black arrows*).

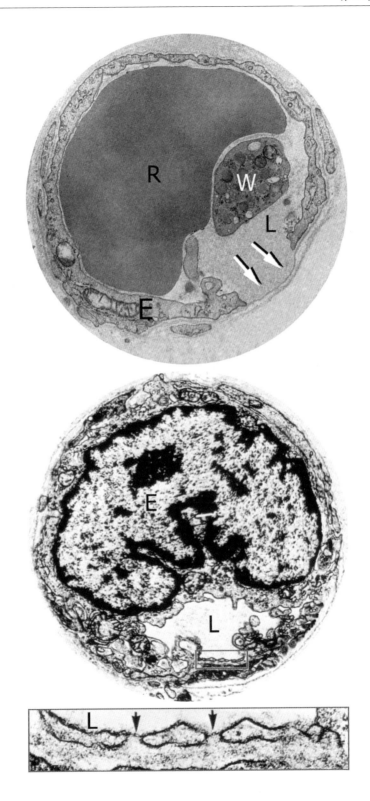

图 37

脉络膜血管的渗透性

> **正常的脉络膜血管允许荧光素透过**。

换句话说,正常的脉络膜血管是"渗漏"的,致使脉络膜背景荧光在荧光血管造影过程中呈弥漫性着染。

这一现象源于脉络膜毛细血管存在微孔(图 38)。

绿箭头=细胞微孔

Permeability of choroidal vessels

> **Normal choroidal vessels are permeable to fluorescein.**

In other words, normal choroidal vessels are "*leaky*". This fact is responsible for the diffuse staining of the background during fluorescein angiography.

The phenomenon is based on the fact that choroidal capillaries have *pores*.

green arrows = pores

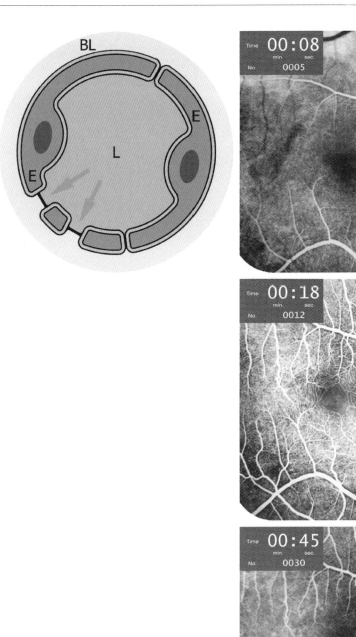

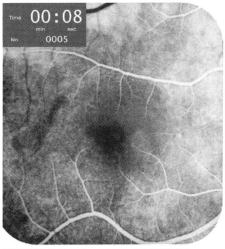

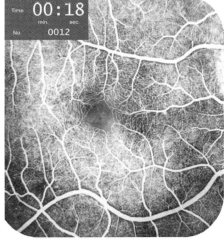

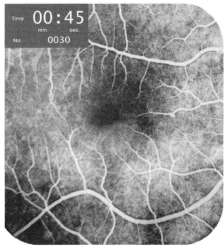

图 38

正常

微孔

> 脉络膜毛细血管壁横切片电镜检查显示内皮细胞存在微孔(图 39)。
>
> 箭头=内皮细胞微孔

Normal

Pores

> Electron microscopic cross sections of walls of choroidal capillaries. The endothelial cells carry
>
> *pores.*
>
> *arrows = pores*

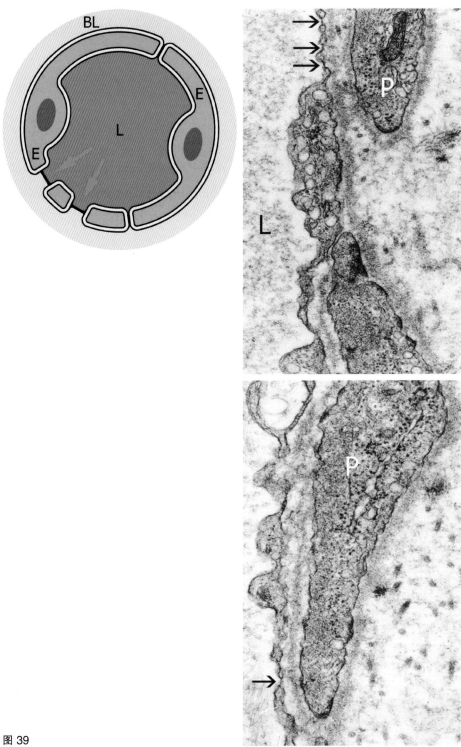

图 39

> 与纵切片(图 40 右上)相比,水平切片电镜检查能更好地显示脉络膜毛细血管内皮细胞微孔的数量及间距(图 40 中及下)。

箭头=微孔

> As compared with perpendicular sections (*top right*), number and spacing of choroidal capillary pores can be appreciated much better on electron microscopic flat sections (*middle and bottom*).

arrow = pore

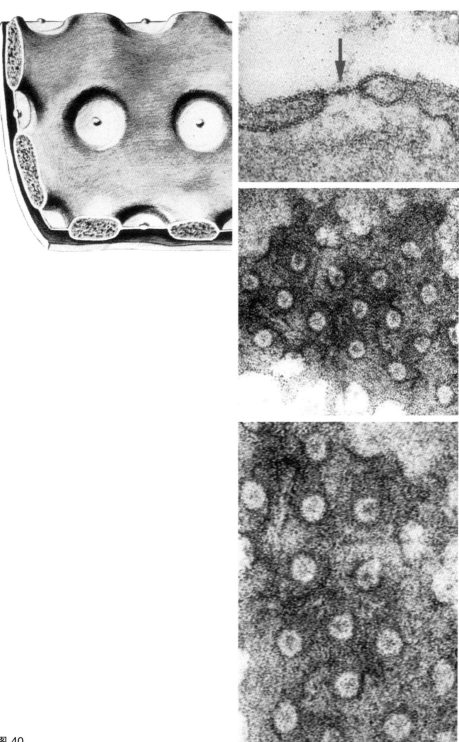

图 40

闭锁小带

❱ 尽管存在细胞微孔,脉络膜内皮细胞间的细胞间隙仍然被闭锁小带所关闭(图41)。

绿箭头=细胞微孔;蓝箭头=闭锁小带

Zonulae occludentes

❱ Despite the presence of pores, the intercellular spaces between the choroidal endothelial cells are closed by *zonulae occludentes*.

green arrows = pores, blue arrows = zonulae occludentes

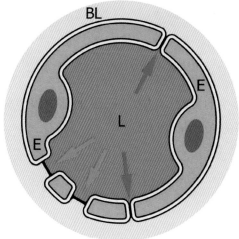

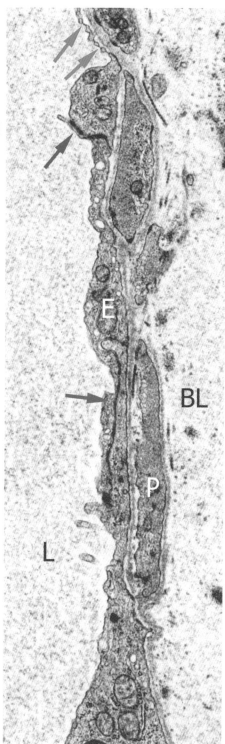

图 41

病理性

> 炎症时,闭锁小带开放。

与通过毛细血管细胞微孔上半通透性膜发生的广泛、有序、"正常"的脉络膜渗漏不同,闭锁小带开放引起渗漏增加,呈局灶性、无序的强渗漏(图 42)。

Pathologic

> Under *inflammatory conditions* the zonulae occludentes open up.

In contrast to the widespread, controlled, "normal" choroidal leakage through the semi-permeable membranes covering the capillary pores, opening of zonulae occludentes causes additional leakage, which is focal, uncontrolled and intense.

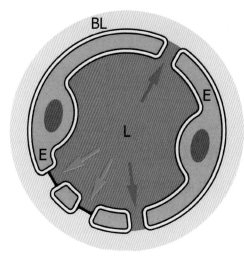

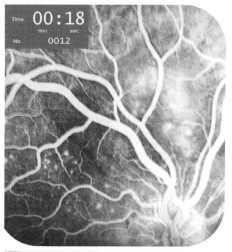

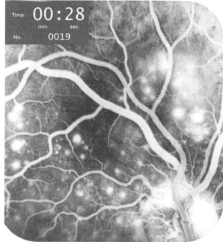

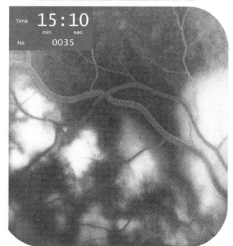

图 42

RPE 的渗透性

正常

闭锁小带

> **正常的 RPE 不允许荧光素通过。**

换句话说,正常的 RPE 连接致密,能阻止荧光素从脉络膜进入神经视网膜。

这主要是因为存在闭锁小带层,封闭了单层色素上皮细胞层全部细胞间隙的顶端部分 (图 43)。

绿箭头=闭锁小带

Permeability of retinal pigment epithelium

Normal

Zonulae occludentes

> **Normal retinal pigment epithelium is non-permeable to fluorescein.**

In other words, normal retinal pigment epithelium is *tight*, thus preventing diffusion of fluorescein from the choroid to the neurosensory retina.

The phenomenon is based on the presence of a layer of *zonulae occludentes* sealing the apical portion of all the intercellular spaces of the pigment epithelial monolayer.

green arrow = zonula occludens

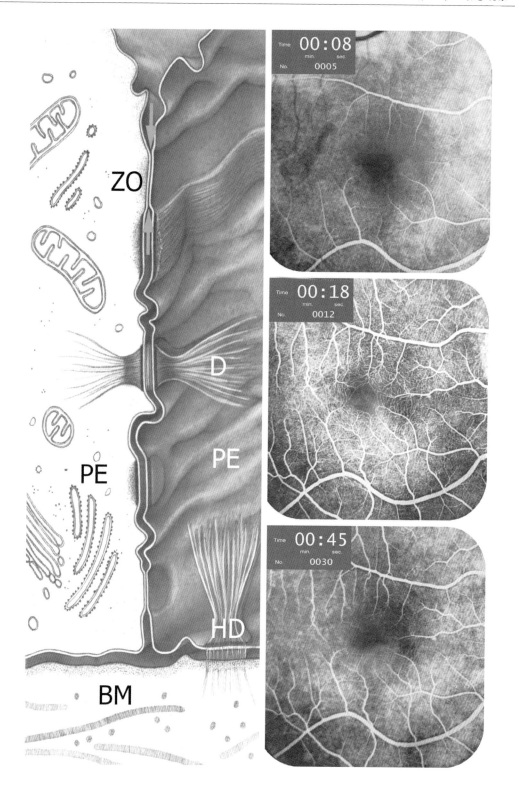

图 43

脉络膜视网膜扩散

❯ 电镜片(图 44)演示了色素上皮屏障阻碍源自脉络膜的扩散。全身注射过氧化物酶后,黑色示踪剂充斥于脉络膜毛细血管中,通过脉络膜毛细血管管壁微孔扩散,并自由迁移通过 Bruch 膜。示踪剂充斥于色素上皮细胞间隙的基底部分(A),但由于受闭锁小带阻碍而停止前行(B),未能到达细胞间隙的顶端部分(C)。

图 44 左上图为荧光素扩散状态的示意图。

Chorioretinal diffusion

❯ The *pigment epithelial barrier* to diffusion originating in the choroid is demonstrated with the electron microscope. After systemic injection of peroxidase, the black tracer material fills the choriocapillaris, diffuses through the pores of the choroidal capillaries, and migrates freely through Bruch's membrane. It fills the basal portion of the pigment epithelial intercellular space (*A*), is stopped by the zonula occludens (*B*), and does not reach the apical portion of the intercellular space (*C*).

The drawing at the *top left* gives an impression of the situation with fluorescein.

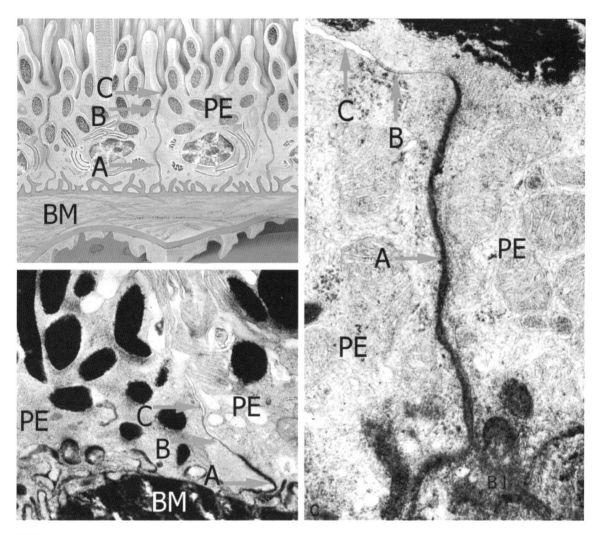

图 44

视网膜脉络膜扩散

❱ 色素上皮闭锁小带同样也不允许源自玻璃体或神经视网膜的扩散(图 45)。黑色示踪剂注入玻璃体腔后,通过神经视网膜扩散进入色素上皮细胞间隙顶端部分(C),并被闭锁小带阻止前行(B)。

因此,细胞间隙基底部分无示踪剂着染(A)。

Retinochorioidal diffusion

❱ The pigment epithelial zonulae occludentes are impermeable also to diffusion originating from the vitreous or the neurosensory retina. Black tracer material injected into the vitreous cavity diffuses through the neurosensory retina and enters the apical portion of the pigment epithelial intercellular space (C), and is stopped by the zonula occludens (B).

Here, the basal portion of the intercellular space (A) remains free of tracer.

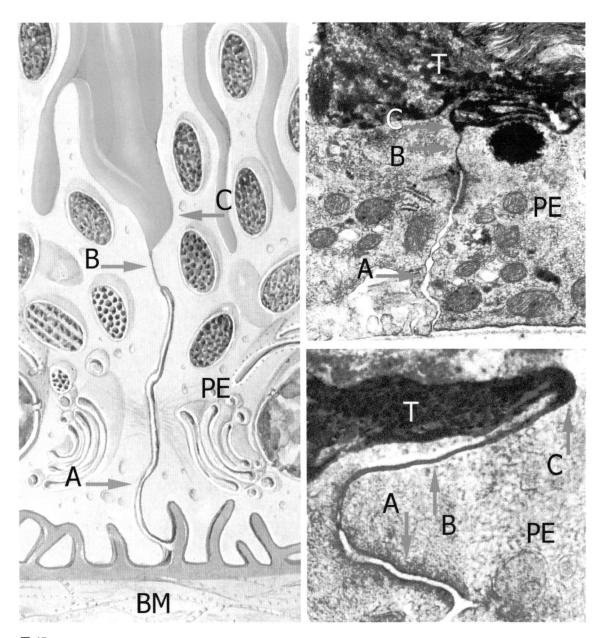

图 45

❯ 总之,RPE 的闭锁小带层代表血-视网膜屏障,阻止了通过细胞微孔,由脉络膜毛细血管漏出的物质(图 46)。而视网膜血管屏障,如前所述,位于血管壁自身(图 30)。

❯ In summary, the layer of zonulae occludentes of the retinal pigment epithelium thus represents the *blood-retinal barrier* for substances circulating through the pore-bearing, leaky choroidal vessels, while for the retinal vessels the barrier is located in the vascular wall itself, as explained previously (*Fig.30*).

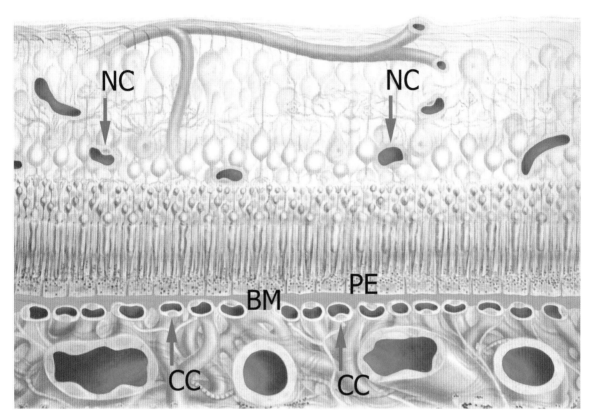

图 46

病理性

瘢痕中的扩散

❯ 正常 RPE 的闭锁小带为扩散的屏障(图 47 左)。

然而,脉络膜视网膜瘢痕缺少闭锁小带,所以缺乏扩散屏障(图 47 右)。因此,激光光凝瘢痕处应该存在开放的细胞间隙,从而可使来自脉络膜的液体积存于其周围的视网膜。但是实际上并没有,其原因将在下节阐述。

Pathologic

Diffusion in scars

❯ *Normal retinal pigment epithelium* with its zonulae occludentes is a *diffusion barrier* (*left*).

However, *chorioretinal scars* lack zonulae occludentes and therefore *are not a diffusion barrier* (*right*). As a result, photocoagulation scars with their open intercellular spaces should lead to an accumulation of choroidal fluid in the surrounding retina, but they do not. The reason for this is explained on the next page.

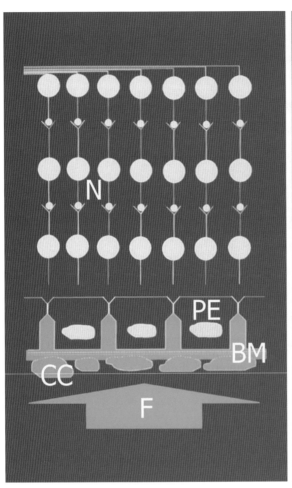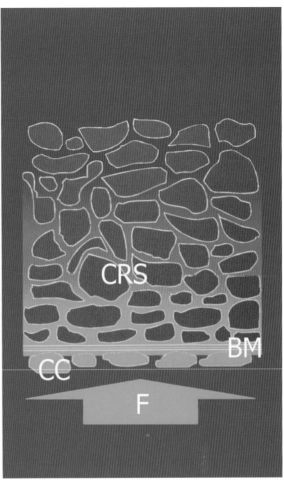

图 47

瘢痕中的液流运动

> 脉络膜毛细血管能吸收液体。

因此,脉络膜视网膜瘢痕中 RPE 屏障的中断产生了视网膜–脉络膜方向的净液流,同时伴有与液流同向的视网膜–脉络膜方向的物质扩散,及反向的脉络膜–视网膜方向的物质扩散(图 48)。

Fluid movement in scars

> Choroidal capillaries *attract fluid*.

Consequently, interruption of the RPE barrier as in chorioretinal scars results in a *net flow of fluid* in a retinochoroidal direction and simultaneously in a *diffusion of substances* in both a retinochoroidal direction, i.e. *with the flow*, and a chorioretinal direction, i.e. *against the flow*.

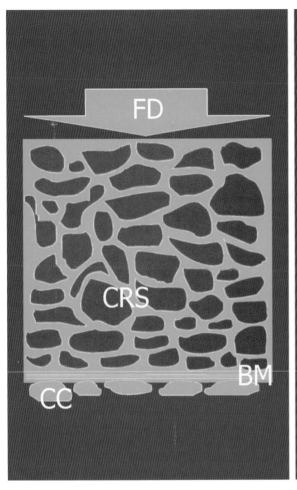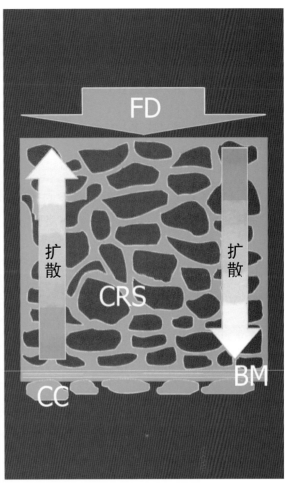

图 48

激光瘢痕

❯ 为进一步说明,图49演示了一脉络膜视网膜激光瘢痕,瘢痕中央部分脉络毛细血管关闭,边缘部分脉络毛细血管开放。

图中荧光小环显示了与液流反向的物质扩散,激光光凝瘢痕周围的脉络膜毛细血管仍保持开放,荧光素渗漏,故着染。

通过色素上皮屏障中断处的视网膜−脉络膜液流运动解释了激光光凝瘢痕如何将神经视网膜内或其下积存的液体排入脉络膜。

Laser scars

❯ For clarification, this is demonstrated again in a graph of a *chorioretinal laser* scar with the closed choriocapillaris in the center and the open choriocapillaris at the edges of the scar.

The *diffusion of material against the stream* is illustrated by the small rim of migrating fluorescein that stains the periphery of photocoagulation scars in the region where the choriocapillaris has remained open.

The retinochoroidal fluid movement across breaks in the pigment epithelial barrier explains why photocoagulation *scars drain fluid accumulations* in, or under, the neurosensory retina into the choroid.

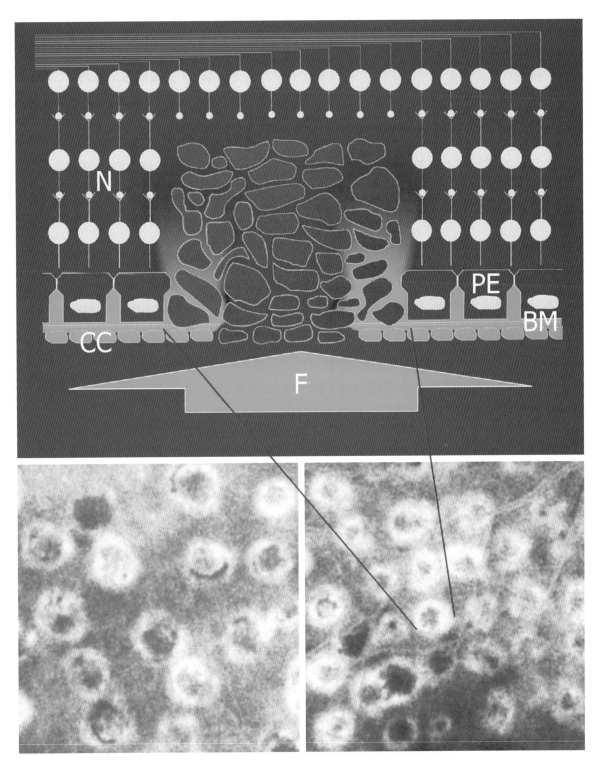

图 49

中心性浆液性脉络膜视网膜病变

❯ 视网膜色素上皮扩散屏障中细小的局限性中断发生于Ⅰ型CSC。通过这个渗漏点,来自脉络膜的液体可以通过色素上皮积聚在神经视网膜下。典型的渗漏特征为渗漏点逐渐扩大(图50)。

由于视网膜色素上皮扩散屏障细小的中断可能导致视网膜–脉络膜方向的液流运动(图38),因此,CSC中脉络膜–视网膜方向大量的液流运动必然是一个更为复杂过程的结果。

Central serous chorioretinopathy

❯ A very small focal breakdown of the retinal pigmenthelial diffusion barrier occurs in the so-called *type I of central serous chorioretinopathy(CSC)*. Through this leakage point fluid from the choroid can cross the pigment epithelium and accumulate under the neurosensory retina. As a typical sign of leakage the leakage point seems to grow.

Since simple breakdown of the pigment epithelial diffusion barrier would lead to fluid movement in retinochoroidal direction (*Fig.38*), the massive fluid movement of CSC in chorioretinal direction must be the result of a more complex process.

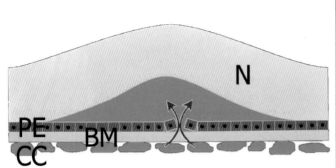

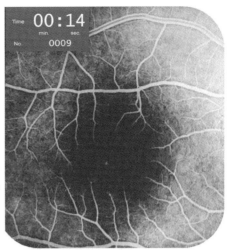

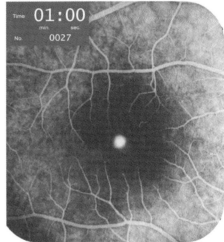

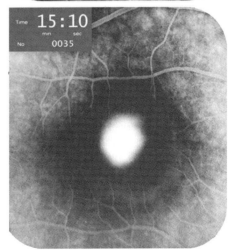

图 50

❯ 在约 6% 的 CSC 病例中,荧光素通过色素上皮渗漏点向上扩散,呈伞样征(图 51)。这一现象又称为"烟窗现象",可能与漏出液和已经积聚在神经视网膜下液体的温度或比重之间存在差异有关。

❯ In about 6% of the cases of central serous chorioretinopathy, the fluorescein passing through the pigment epithelial leakage point moves upwards and may spread in an umbrella-like fashion. This finding, the so-called *smoke-stack phenomenon*, is said to be related to differences in either the temperature or the specific weight between the leaking fluid and the liquid that has already accumulated under the neurosensory retina.

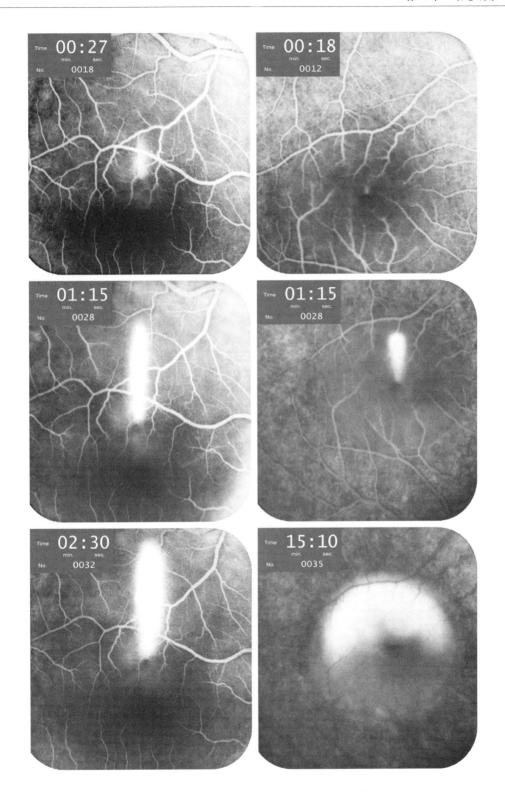

图 51

❯ 正常的 RPE 主动吸收视网膜-脉络膜方向的液流,这一功能通过某些离子运动实现。这意味着,RPE 或者下方脉络膜在某种机制不明的损伤过程的影响下,小部分 RPE 细胞,甚至可能仅是个别细胞发生了功能逆转,向脉络膜-视网膜方向分泌大量离子,即分泌至神经视网膜下腔,由此吸引脉络膜的液流进入该区域。最初,必定发生了跨细胞的液流运动。然而,过强的液流可能导致相应区域的 RPE 中断,有时甚至使得周围的 RPE 细胞基底部从 Bruch 膜分离。由于色素上皮缺损区域极其微小,因此在荧光血管造影早期,仅可见针尖样渗漏点(图 52)。

❯ *Normal retinal pigment epithelium* actively *absorbs* fluid in a retinochoroidal direction. This is accomplished by the movement of certain ions. It is conceivable that, under the influence of an as yet undefined damaging process in the pigment epithelium or the underlying choroid, a minute group of RPE cells, possibly even a single cell, reverses its function and *secretes* large amounts of ions in chorioretinal direction, i.e. into the subneuroretinal space, thus attracting choroidal fluid into this area. Initially, the fluid movement certainly occurs transcellularly. The flow is so strong, however, that it possibly disrupts the pigment epithelium in the involved area and sometimes even detaches the base of the surrounding RPE cells from Bruch's membrane. Since the defective area of pigment epithelium is very small, only a tiny leakage point is visible during the earliest phase of fluorescein angiography.

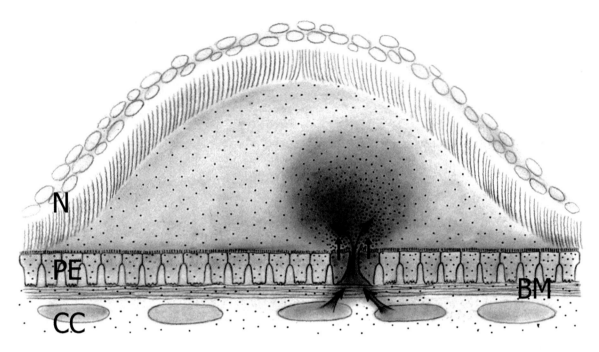

图 52

> 视网膜下积液并不渗漏荧光素进入周围的视网膜及玻璃体。这可能是因为积液周围的细胞间隙被新形成的紧密连接所封闭,就和发生在其他视网膜积液的情况一样。

可以肯定的是,通过渗漏点进入积液腔的液体又被渗漏点附近的色素上皮细胞泵回了脉络膜。治愈后,作为这一应激反应的结果是,原神经上皮脱离灶下方整个区域受累的细胞,出现持久性的色素紊乱。

> The *subretinal blister does not leak* fluorescein into the surrounding retina and from there into the vitreous. It is likely that the intercellular spaces surrounding the blister are sealed off by newly formed tight junctions as they occur in other retinal fluid accumulations.

It is safe to conclude that the fluid that enters the blister through the leakage point is *pumped back* into the choroid by the pigment epithelial cells neighboring the leakage point. After healing and as a consequence of the stress, the cells involved show a lasting pigmentary disturbance in the entire area underlying the former neurosensory detachment.

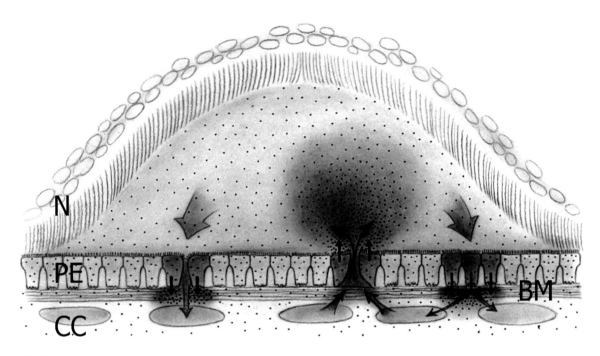

图 53

❯ Ⅲ型 CSC 是前两型的复合型,既存在色素上皮的脱离(见图 27),也存在神经上皮的脱离(见图 50)。渗漏点可以在色素上皮脱离灶内(图 54a),也可以在色素上皮脱离灶外(图 54b)。

血管造影时,在色素上皮脱离区没有染料渗漏,仅表现为荧光积存,且着染区大小不变(图 54 星号),而色素上皮渗漏点逐渐扩大(图 54 箭头)。

❯ *Type* Ⅲ *central serous chorioretinopathy* is a combination of the two previous types comprising *both* a pigment epithelial detachment (*Fig.27*) *and* a neurosensory detachment (*Fig.50*) with a leakage point located within (*a*) or outside (*b*) the area of pigment epithelial detachment.

The angiogram of such a condition reveals only pooling and no leakage of dye in the area of pigment epithelial detachment and the stained area does not change its size (*asterisk*), whereas the leakage point in the pigment epithelium seems to grow (*arrow*).

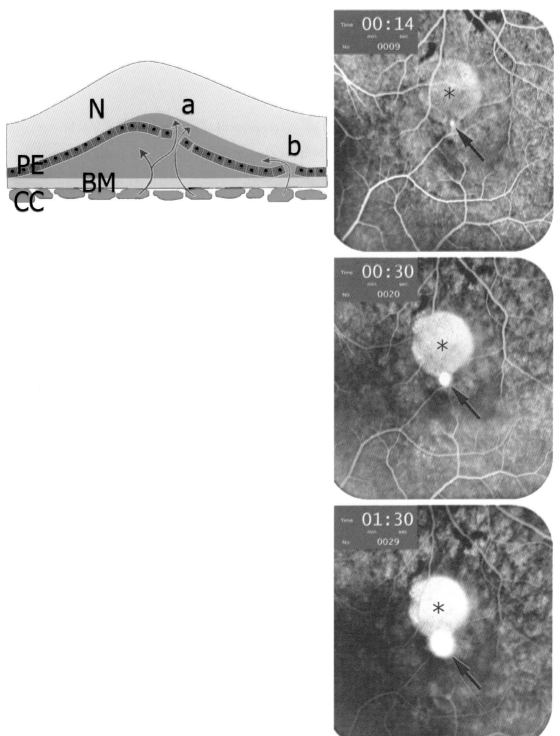

图 54

> 混合型的小渗漏点(图 55 红箭头)伴神经视网膜下大量积液(图 55 十字),及其下方小的色素上皮脱离(图 55 白箭头,图 55 星号)均可在 OCT 上清晰地显示(图 55 左)。

> The combination of a small leakage point(*red arrow*) with a large subneuroretinal blister (*cross*) overlying a small pigment epithelial detachment (*white arrow*, *asterisk*) is nicely demonstrated also on OCT (*left*).

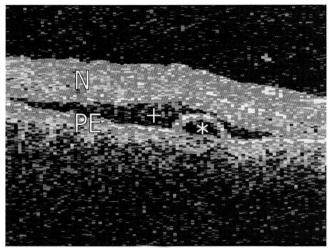

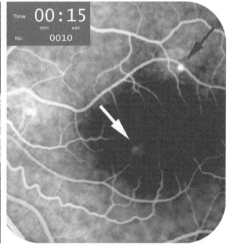

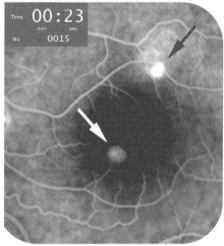

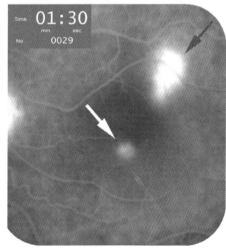

图 55

年龄相关性黄斑变性

▶ 脉络膜新生血管(choroidal neovascularizations,CNV)见于多种疾病,也可以引起 RPE 脱离(见图 27)和(或)神经视网膜脱离(见图 50)。

当新生血管位于 RPE 下时(图 56a),其可见度依赖于上方覆盖的 RPE 色素颗粒的数量。然而,当新生血管突破色素上皮进入神经视网膜下间隙(图 56b)时,其可见度取决于神经视网膜透明度。在图 56 的病例中,新生血管周围的暗环是由于出血遮蔽荧光所致(图 56 右)。

Age-related macular degeneration

▶ Detachment of the retinal pigment epithelium (*Fig.27*) and/or the neurosensory retina (*Fig.50*) can be caused also by *choroidal neovascularizations* which are found in a variety of conditions. When the proliferated vessels lie below the retinal pigment epithelium(*a*)their visibility depends on the amount of pigment granules in the overlying retinal pigment epithelium; however,when the newly formed vessels extend through the pigment epithelium into the subneuroretinal space (*b*),they are visible due to the transparency of the neurosensory retina. The dark ring surrounding the proliferated vessels in the case presented on the opposite page is created by blood that blocks underlying fluorescence.

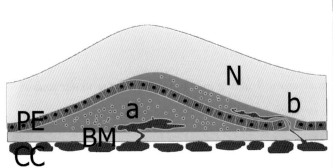

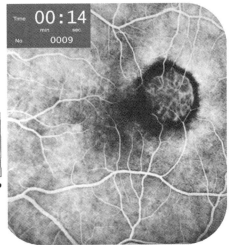

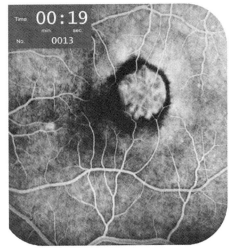

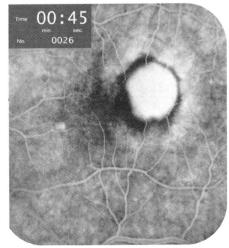

图 56

> 新形成的脉络膜血管突破 Bruch 膜,长入 RPE 下或上,形成血管网,类似于脉络膜毛细血管(图 57)。

> The newly formed choroidal vessels that cross Bruch's membrane and grow *under and/or over* the retinal pigment epithelium form a *network imitating the choriocapillaris*(Fig.57).

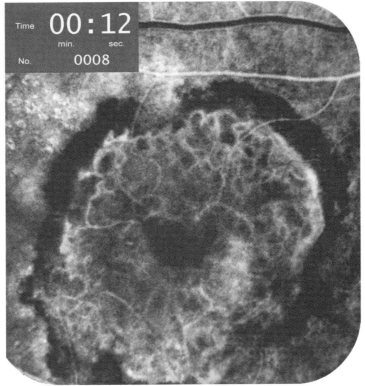

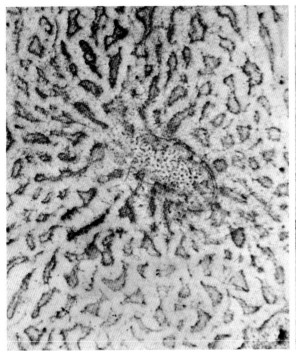

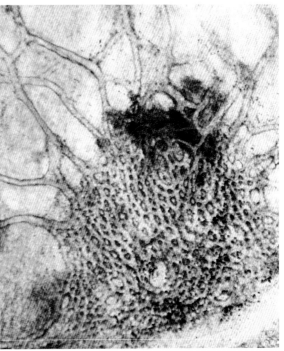

图 57

❭ 与其来源的脉络膜血管相似,新生的血管也存在微孔,因此渗漏荧光素(图 58)。

❭ Like the choroidal vessels they originate from, the proliferated vessels have *pores* and therefore leak fluorescein(Fig.58).

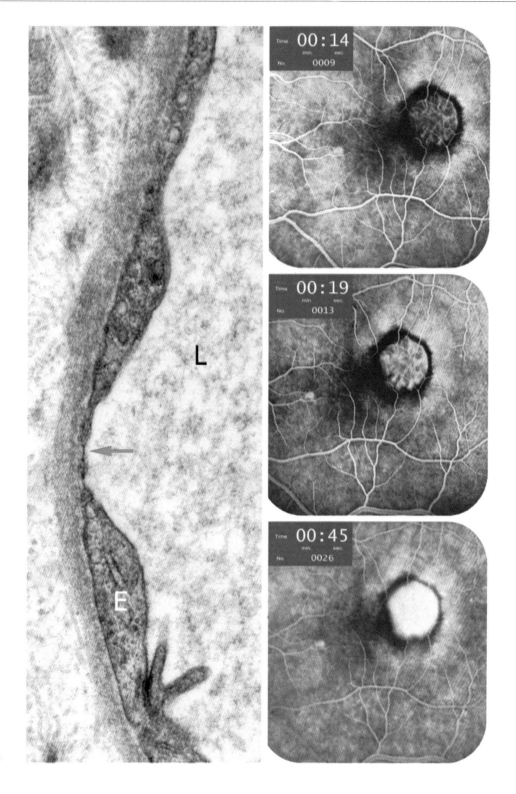

图 58

图片参考文献

Figure References

图1下、图2下、图3上、图44左上、图45左、图46改编自：

Wiederholt M，Bräuer H，Bräuer B（1999）Mikrozirkulation des Auges. Medical Service München（MSM），Munich

图5下、图13下，图22、图23引自：

Spitznas M（1974）

The fine structure of the chorioretinal border tissues of the adult human eye. Advances in Ophthalmology 28:78–174，Karger，Basel

图26上，图43左改编自：

Hogan M，Alvarado J，Wedell J（1971）

Histology of the human eye. Saunders，Philadelphia

图18上改编自：

Pauleikoff D，Münster，Germany

图29上左、上中改编自：

Rhodin JAG（1962）Journal of Ultrastructure Research 6:171–185，Academic Press

附　录
Appendix

BL	basal lamina	基底膜
BM	Bruch's membrane	Bruch 膜
CC	choriocapillaris	脉络膜毛细血管
CRS	chorioretinal scar	脉络膜视网膜瘢痕
D	desmosome	桥粒
E	endothelial cell	内皮细胞
F	fluorescein	荧光素
FD	fluid	液流
FL	fusion line	融合线
HD	hemidesmosome	半桥粒
M	melanin granule	黑色素颗粒
N	neurosensory retina	神经视网膜
NC	retinal capillary	视网膜毛细血管
OS	outer segments	外节
P	pericyte	周细胞
RPE	retinal pigment epithelium	视网膜色素上皮
R	red blood cell	红细胞
T	tracer material	示踪剂
V	villous processes	绒毛
W	white blood cell	白细胞
Z	zonula occludens	闭锁小带